<u>**Disclaimer Notice:**</u>

Please note the information contained within this document is for educational and entertainment purposes only. Every attempt has been made to provide accurate, up to date and reliable complete information. No warranties of any kind are expressed or implied. Readers acknowledge that the author is not engaging in the rendering of legal, financial, medical or professional advice.

By reading this document, the reader agrees that under no circumstances are we responsible for any losses, direct or indirect, which are incurred as a result of the use of information contained within this document, including, but not limited to, —errors, omissions, or inaccuracies.

TABLE OF CONTENTS

Introduction

Due to the damaging impacts of negative behaviors, countless articles and books have been written on how to identify them, their triggers, and how to overcome them. There is no doubt that these efforts are commendable, and many people have been able to improve the quality of their lives by leveraging the tips in these materials. However, the fact that many writers and readers fail to see is that bad behavior is essentially the absence of healthy ones. Therefore, if good habits can be promoted, they will automatically eliminate and replace destructive ones.

This conviction is the reason behind this project. Health is the most important thing in this world. Sadly, many people don't realize it until they lose it. The reality is that our health will deteriorate as we grow older and move towards the end of our lives. Nonetheless, we can choose to age gradually or look older than our real age due to poor health management. Healthy habits ensure that you will be able to stay more away from the doctor and have the strength to carry out your daily activities.

It is high time you prioritized your health. If you are sick, it is going to be difficult for you to achieve and live your dreams. Your loved ones need you to be healthy. If your physical health is affected, it will affect every other aspect of your life including your mental and social health. Life becomes colorless and meaningless when you are not healthy. What is the way out? Leverage the tips in this book.

Chapter 1: What are Healthy Habits?

It is logical to start this book by investigating healthy habits. Indeed, they are numerous. So, we will highlight the characteristics of healthy habits and remind you about what really matters the most in life.

What Matters the Most in Life

In the midst of the craze and rush of the modern world, many people forget the most important things in life. Many never learn to value those things until they lose them. It is this lack of getting our priorities right that is responsible for the rate of depression in the world today. Many people are unhappy despite the money and achievements they have. They keep wondering what is missing. The answer is not farfetched. They have forgotten how to live.

Here are some of the most important things in life that many people neglect.

Loved Ones

The desire to be rich and famous has made many people forget that it's lonely at the top when you're not there with your loved ones. Some people cry on the days they receive awards because they wish their friends, families, and any other person that matters to them were present. In reality, there are some situations in which we lose our loved ones to accidents.

However, in some cases, they leave us because we are selfish and don't have regard for them. We are busy chasing our dreams while making them feel that they take secondary places in our lives. King Midas, in ancient Greek mythology, learned the hard way that no amount of treasure in this world could replace his daughter. You don't have to lose your loved ones before you figure that out.

Happiness

Happiness is the greatest pursuit of man, even though many people don't realize it. The reason you want to chase and live your dream is that you want to be happy. Sadly, many people get all they want only to realize that they don't want what they got. In other words, they chased the big life because they thought it would make them happy only to realize that they felt hollow and empty after achieving their targets.

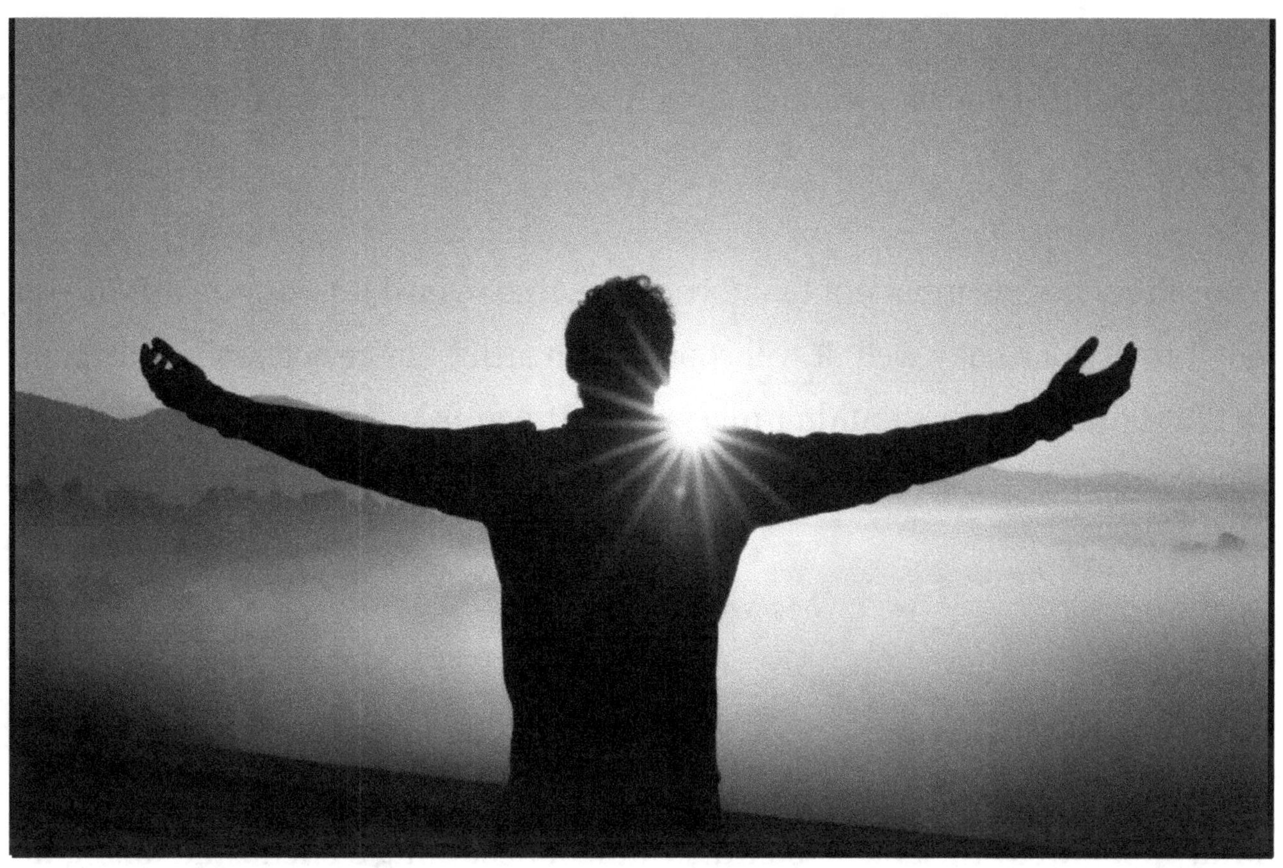

You don't have to possess a private jet or wear expensive clothes to be happy. Enjoying the camaraderie of your loved ones is enough to make you happy. The issue is that many people have friends that don't value them because of the things they don't possess. Still, if you find yourself among people who love and respect you regardless of what you have, you will understand that happiness is in the simple things of life.

Health

Note that health is not simply the absence of diseases, according to the World Health Organization. It also refers to your mental and social life. Your health is very crucial to the quality of life you live. It is harder to be happy or enjoy the company of your loved ones when you are sick. So, you should never toy with it.

Your job schedule must not make you have less regard for your health. If you don't treat your body well, it will soon "go on strike" or "evict you". Your body is that landlord you shouldn't mess with. It wants to be respected, and you will wake up to a rude shock when you aren't doing what you ought to do.

Health is Wealth

Many people say the above maxim is almost becoming a cliché and losing its relevance. Nevertheless, it remains an important truthful statement that you can only treat with levity at your own peril. Health is wealth and there is no doubt about that. At least, you need it to make wealth. You cannot go to work if you are sick unless it is very minor. Even when it is minor, you will still find it difficult to be at your best when you don't have sound health.

Moreover, you need to be healthy to enjoy your success. What is the point of making all the money only to spend it on sickness? You should take an "excursion" to the hospital once in a while to learn some vital lessons in life. There are many rich people in the hospital who are there battling for their lives. They have money but they don't have the sound health that money cannot buy.

The fact that you can afford an expensive meal doesn't mean that you should buy it. You should consider the health implications of the things you consume rather than their prices. Success is only worth it when you are in good health and can enjoy it with the people that mean the world to you.

What Makes a Habit Healthy?

We will end this section by identifying the qualities of healthy habits in order to help you identify them and avoid destructive ones. Healthy habits have the following attributes.

Beneficial to the Individual in the Long Run

It is crucial to mention that a habit should be beneficial in the long run before it can be considered to be healthy. There are many things we do that gratify our desires in the short run but are disastrous in the long run. For example, smoking settles the desire to feel calm in the short run. However, it affects the lung and other parts of the body eventually.

So, if a habit cannot make you stay healthy in the long run, you shouldn't let the short-term benefits blindfold you. Lack of consideration for the future consequences of an action will only bring tears and regrets eventually.

Beneficial to Others

When something is beneficial to you but hurts others, it's not a good habit. We have to be conscious about how our actions affect the people around us. This is the reason the government of some nations restricts the activities of industries. The fact that a company is boosting the economy and raking in a lot of money doesn't mean it has the freedom to jeopardize our health.

We should apply the same principle when evaluating our habits. For example, sexual promiscuity might make you feel good immediately. Nonetheless, it will hurt your partner emotionally when he or she finds out. In some cases, it might even affect the person physically if you infect him or her with sexually transmitted diseases from unprotected sex.

Beneficial to your Physical and Mental Health

It's in your best interest to consider how your actions affect both your physical and mental health. If a habit affects your mental health negatively, it will eventually take its toll on your physical health, and vice versa. So, the fact that an action doesn't have a direct impact on your physical health doesn't mean it is right for you. For example, you might be doing a job that doesn't demand too much from you physically. Nonetheless, if you are told to do unethical things that don't align with your conscience, you'll not be happy.

The feeling of dissatisfaction will become more intense when you realize that your activities are hurting people. If you keep having negative emotions, it can affect the way you take care of your physical health. For example, when you're not in a good mood, it's not likely that you have an appetite. The desire to exercise or enjoy sex if you are married might become affected. So, a good habit doesn't only have physical health benefits; it should also have mental health advantages.

Chapter 2: Lifestyle Choices

Life is a game of choices, and you have to choose wisely. We should never forget that we have the right to pick our choices but we don't have the right to decide the consequences of our decisions.

Making the Best Personal Decisions

The quality of your life depends on the quality of your choices. Whatever you're experiencing today is often a product of your previous investments. You don't have to wait until you are sick before you start eating healthily and working out. You can choose to have a culture of having a healthy lifestyle to protect your health both in the short-term and long run. Note that you are always making a decision even when it seems as though you're not doing anything. Indecision and choosing to do nothing are still choices.

You should be more deliberate about the choices you make because they all have consequences, which can be either positive or negative. For example, you shouldn't just eat anything you can grab. It's a wrong approach to feeding that can make you gain excess weight or jeopardize your health. An adage says, "You are what you eat". Regardless of your perception of this statement, it's not far from the truth.

Your choice of food and how you eat it affect several parts of your life, including your physique and overall health. Nonetheless, your feeding habit isn't the only lifestyle choice you make. Your choice to commit to a daily workout or the decision to stay off will also bring its consequences.

Lifestyle Choices

A lifestyle choice refers to a personal and deliberate decision to carry out a behavior that may decrease or increase the risk of disease or injury. It's likely that you have made lifestyle choices already. For example, if you have decided to take a walk for thirty minutes every day, it is a lifestyle choice. In the same way, if you have made the decision to stay away from alcohol, it is a lifestyle choice that will promote your wellbeing and help you avoid damaging consequences.

By deciding to avoid or reduce alcohol consumption, you are decreasing the chances of a car crash due to driving while drunk. You're also reducing the risk of liver damage when you make this choice. Ultimately, you are decreasing the chances of dying early. Besides, the stigma that comes with being known as an alcoholic can take its toll on your mental health.

Unhealthy Lifestyle Choices

Most of the lifestyle choices that have been mentioned so far are positive. However, there are negative ones too. They can cause devastating damages to the person that has this lifestyle and also the people around them. Below are examples of unhealthy lifestyle choices.

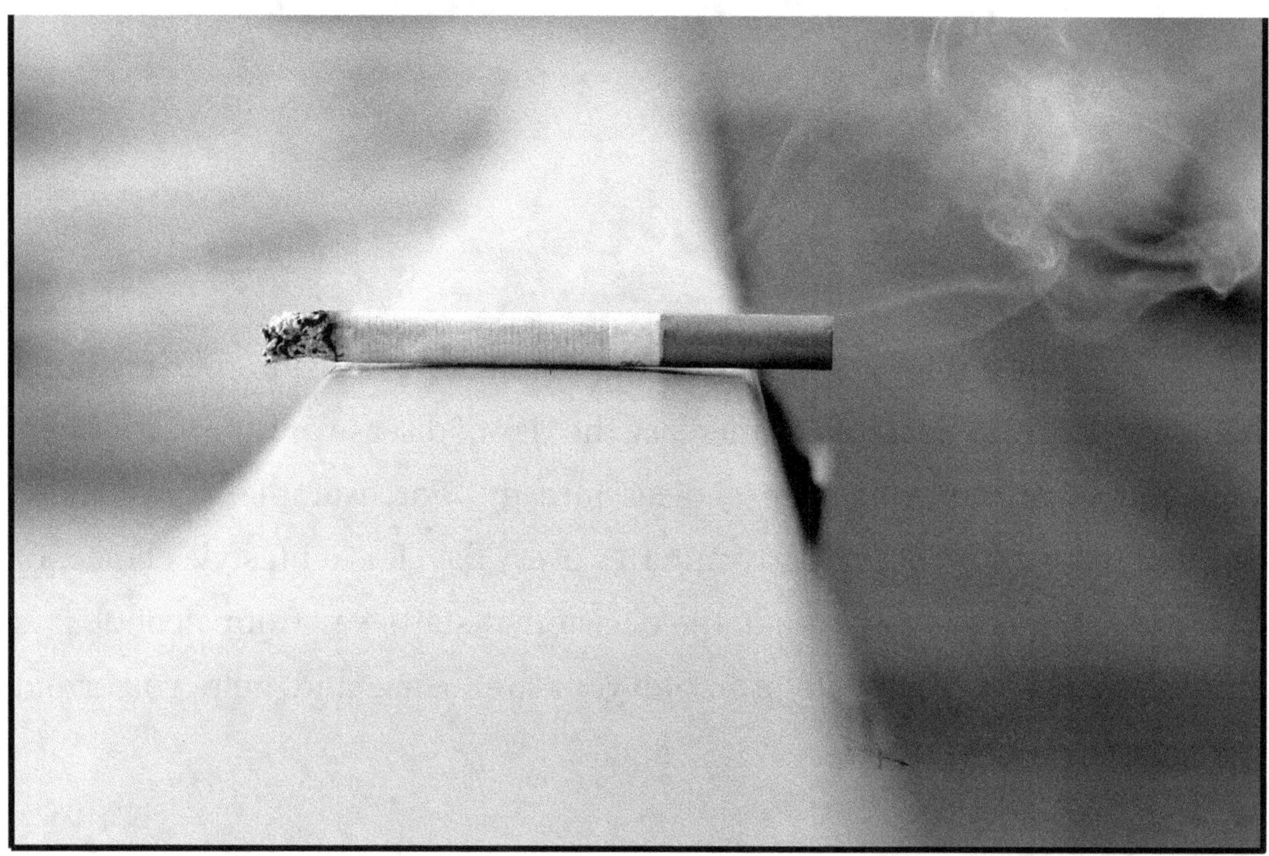

Smoking

An example of a negative lifestyle choice is smoking. It is a major risk factor for different cancers, including lung cancer. Smoking doesn't only affect the smoker; it also has destructive impacts on the people around the smoker. For example, the individuals around a smoker are also inhaling the smoke coming from the cigarette. So, they end up suffering the same or even worse health issues. If you smoke, you're not the only one at risk. The people around you are also at risk because they are passive smokers.

Use of Firearms

The use of a firearm is also a dangerous lifestyle choice. It's not safe, especially if you have issues with anger management. You could hurt others and also yourself on a day when you are frustrated. Indeed, it can help in self-defense, especially in states where they are legal. Nonetheless, you should think twice before you procure one even if you are living in that kind of location. The fact that something is legal doesn't mean it is good for you. Seek other alternatives that can help you apart from it.

Drug Abuse

If you have a habit of taking drugs without a doctor's prescription or supervision, you are also playing a dangerous game. Drugs are chemical substances. Therefore, when you consume them, they will affect your body in ways you might never know. Most drugs have side effects. It's only that some are mild. Still, some drugs have devastating side effects ranging from pregnancy complications to constipation.

Some drugs, especially heroin and cannabis, can lead to addiction problems. They can also cause hallucinations, thereby interfering with your ability to perform your daily tasks. So, it is in your best interest to avoid experimenting with drugs. Doctors and other professional medical experts are trained to understand the content of medications and their effects. Therefore, it is in your best interest to trust their judgment when choosing to take or leave a drug.

How to Break Free from Harmful Habits

The best way to break free from harmful habits is to avoid them. Prevention is always better than cure. Once you have started indulging in a habit, it becomes very difficult to stop it. Your body likes it when you have a habit because it increases its efficiency. However, wrong lifestyle choices can have devastating consequences. Therefore, you have to stop them. It's challenging to break free from a negative habit. Nevertheless, it's possible.

One of the best ways you can turn things around is by replacing them with the right ones. For example, instead of smoking or drinking alcohol, you can find other ways to relax or take your mind away from the troubles of life. You can replace these habits with regular workouts or find a hobby. A hobby can improve your mood and make you excited such that you will not need the high that cannabis offers.

Be strategic about choosing a good habit to replace a negative one. If you choose an activity that doesn't offer you the perks you enjoy from an unhealthy habit, the impact isn't likely to last. For example, you cannot replace a bad habit that makes you calm with a good one that makes you excited. You'll still have the craving for calmness, and you may end up going back to the former unhealthy lifestyle choice. So, take your time to ensure that you make a decision that will stand the test of time.

Chapter 3: Work-Life Balance

The Covid-19 pandemic was an unprecedented disaster. It didn't only kill people and cause immeasurable pain to families that lost their loved ones; it also crumbled the economies of many nations. However, it taught many people vital lessons. One of those lessons will be discussed in full detail in this section.

What is Work-Life Balance?

Work-life balance refers to the state of equilibrium where an individual makes the best out of both his or her career and personal life. In other words, it is an arrangement that enables you to move up the ladder of your career without sacrificing your personal relationships. This structure is fast becoming the new norm because of its numerous benefits.

The pandemic made many people realized what they have been missing for so long: work-life balance. Many companies were forced to ask their workers to work from home. It occurred to many people that they will prefer to continue with that arrangement. The chance to work from home is increasingly a preferred option for millennials because it offers work-life balance.

According to a survey by Accel and Qualtrics, 66%percent of millennials are willing to take a pay-cut to work remotely. This shows that many employees are frustrated with their struggles with work-life balance in a traditional team. Working from home enables you to execute projects without having to work from a designated desk. So, it is not surprising that many companies are working with a remote workforce. This approach enables them to get the best out of their employees.

Benefits of Work-Life Balance

Many people only get to do the things they like to do after their retirement. However, some people are getting the best out of life while working because they have a work-life balance. Below are some of the benefits of this lifestyle.

Less Stress

According to a Stanford professor, Jeffrey Pfeffer, workplace stress is killing Americans. In fact, it is rated as the 5th biggest cause of death in the US. Work stress refers to the result of conditions like high job demands, little autonomy on the job, and long hours of working. It damages productivity and morale.

However, it has been discovered to also have a drastic impact on wellbeing. Also, a quarter of Americans believe that their jobs are their main source of stress. Work-life balance helps to reduce stress and increase productivity.

Clear Boundaries

One of the reasons people struggle to have a balance between their career and personal life is due to the lack of clear boundaries between the two. Many people bring their jobs to the house and take their personal life to their workplaces. In other words, many people are guilty of straining their personal relationships by bringing in the pressure they are facing in their office. Also, they talk to their colleagues at work about their families, thereby bothering them with things that ought to stay at home. Work-life balance helps to create boundaries that will help you to have the best of the two worlds.

Improved Mental Health

When you feel that you have no choice but to work yourself out until you are mentally exhausted daily, it will eventually affect your mental health. You feel like a slave that has to do everything possible to make ends meet. Without work-life balance, you are susceptible to negative emotions. You will lack the resources to handle them because you are emotionally overwhelmed.

Enhance Physical Health

Work-life balance doesn't only improve your mental health; it also enhances your physical health. When you have the necessary equilibrium in your career and personal life, you will be more relaxed and create time for more productive activities. You will be able to cook your meal, thereby eating healthily. You will also be able to have healthy sleeping habits and create more time for exercise. The product of these beneficial habits is sound physical health.

Boost Mindfulness

Working too much will strain your personal relationships. If you are married with kids, your spouse and children will feel that your job matters more to you than them. You will hardly have time to see your kids represent their schools or do any other thing that matters to them. The absence of a work-life balance is one of the reasons some marriages that started well broke down and eventually deteriorated into divorces.

Your spouse wants your attention, and he or she may not be able to cope when he or she is not getting it. When you are working moderately, you'll be able to be more present in the moment. You will be able to sit with your loved ones and enjoy their company without interference.

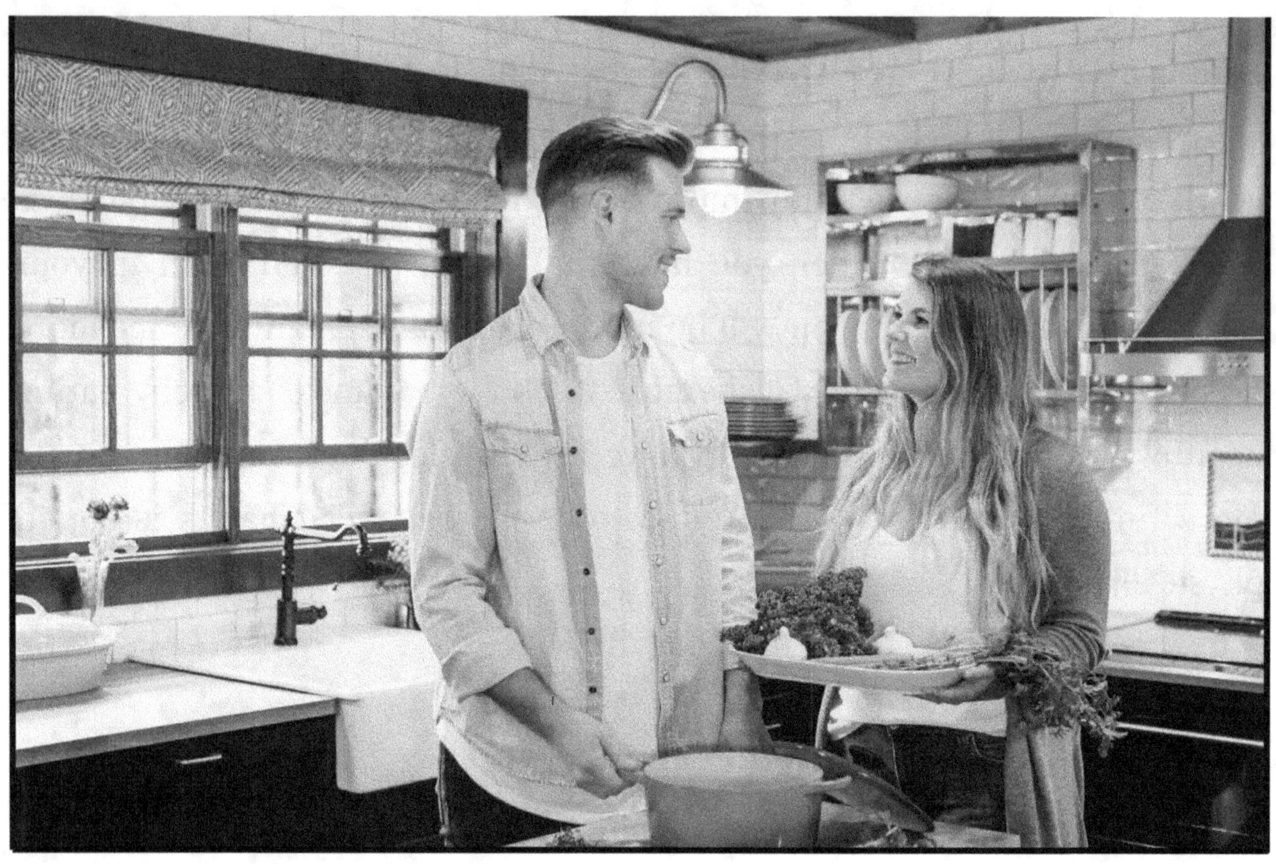

How to Slow Down in the Modern World

It's not good enough to understand the benefits of work-life balance; you should know how to incorporate it. Below are some tips that will help you in this regard.

Discard Perfectionism

The tendency for perfectionism is usually developed at a young age for many overachievers. They put a lot of pressure on themselves to have high performance because the demands on their time are still limited. Sadly, many carry this mindset into adulthood. Their desire to fulfill their potential leads them to an overdrive such that they are willing to neglect other aspects of their lives to climb the ladder of career success. They have been A-grade students, and now, they want to be A-grade workers. This desperation will not let you have a balanced career and personal life.

Reduce the Use of your Digital Devices

It is easier for people to bring their jobs home or take them wherever they go today, thanks to the advent of technology. It's a great advantage because it allows companies to offer more flexibility to their employees. Nonetheless, the problem is that some people don't know how to draw the boundaries because they have access to their workplace right from home. Some are fond of working on their laptops when their spouse and kids are seeking their attention. Have a principle of closing your laptop and keeping your phone away when speaking to your loved ones.

Regular Exercise

Many books and articles have been written about the numerous benefits of regular exercise. Virtually everyone knows its importance. Still, many people have a culture of eliminating it when they are busy. Exercise puts you in a meditative state that brings calmness to your body, according to the Mayo Clinic. No matter how busy you are, you still find time to eat because it is important. You should also treat exercise that way.

Get your Priorities Right

Make a list of the most important things to you in the order of their importance. This list cannot be the same for everyone. Nonetheless, your family, health, and job should be closer to the top. You need this list to recognize some other activities you devote your time to that are time-wasting. The reason some people struggle to have a work-life balance is that they spend excessive time on social media. Identify those activities that waste your time and limit them or eliminate them to create more time for your family and job.

Delegate More

Delegating doesn't only benefit you; it also gives room for others to grow and become more competent. As a career woman, you might need to sit down with your husband and discuss little areas where he can be of help at home to reduce the stress of fixing dinner for the home. Many men will gladly help out if you present the idea to them with the right approach. You can also engage your kids as they grow older.

Chapter 4: Getting the Best out of your Daily Routines

A day lost is a gift you can never regain. Therefore, it is imperative that you enjoy every day of your life as though it might be your last. Remember that what determines the quality of your day is the way you go about your activity. So, you need to change the way you go about the day to get the best out of it. Below are some hacks that can make a difference in your daily routines.

Focus on the Meaning or Benefits

One of the reasons we aren't motivated when carrying out some tasks is that we forget the benefits of that activity somewhere along the line. Indeed, some tasks could be physically demanding, such as doing laundry, mopping, or mowing the yard. Nevertheless, they are not meaningless activities. We carry them out because they are important to our health and the appearance of our home. No one wants to be in a home with overgrown grasses, dusty floors, and stinking clothes. Besides, you don't want your visitors to perceive you as a dirty person.

So, you should use the purpose of the activities as the motivation to complete them without grumbling. One of the reasons you procrastinate is that you have taken your eyes off the essence of the task. Remember how neat and tidy you will look while ironing your clothes. In the same way, think about the personal feeling of satisfaction and good remarks you will get from guests when you clean your home. It's true that you'll feel tired when carrying out the activity, but you will forget all the stress you have gone through when you have completed it.

Make them Fun

Think of innovative ways you can carry out your daily routines to motivate you to do them. For example, you can make using the TV remote, brushing your teeth, and lifting an object more challenging by using your non-preferred hand. Checking your new email can also become a boring routine task despite its importance if you don't seek more effective ways to go about it. You can consider leveraging filters on your Gmail account, which enables you to prioritize some emails. Also, you can consider taking a new route when going to work or returning.

Your mind loves it when you do something in a different way. You can consider turning a routine into a game. For example, you can start checking how long it takes you to make your bed. Then set a challenge to beat that time the next time. You can do this for other activities too. We all love challenges and competitions because they have a way of making us work harder and more efficiently. Even if there is no one to compete with you, you can set up personal challenges that will get you up to speed.

Be at the Center

An activity takes a new look when you pay more attention to details. For example, you can enjoy eating your meal more when you eat slowly and pay attention to the taste of every bite and chunk. If you made the meal, think about the process involved and how your cooking skills have produced that magic. If it is a restaurant, appreciate the technique of the cooks and imagine the energy they put into making the meal. You'll realize that it feels different, unlike when you are just eating for the sake of it.

You can also make the best of your routines when you are present at the moment. Don't read a newspaper when watching a movie. Choose one task at a time and focus on it until you're through. When speaking to people, don't use your phone without seeking their permission. The human mind is not designed to focus on more than one task at a time. When you try to do more than one thing at the same time, you find yourself stressed out. You'll end up not making the best out of any of those activities.

Optimize your Strength

You cannot enjoy your life to the fullest when you haven't discovered yourself. You should know your strengths and weaknesses. When you identify the things you are good at, you will find them enjoyable. Delegate the things you are not fantastic at doing to others, especially when you can afford to pay for extra hands. If mowing the yard ruins your week or day, and you can afford to pay someone else to do it, why not? It doesn't make you lazy. You are only smart enough to concentrate your energy on more productive things.

If you haven't discovered the things you do effortlessly, you will struggle with efficiency. Note that the fact that you're struggling with a task doesn't mean that you're not cut out for it. You might need more training and guidance to do it better. So, ensure you do your research to improve your efficiency. When you are better at doing something, you will find it more fun to do it. You'll stop procrastinating and do more within the time limit you have. Otherwise, you'll keep giving yourself ten reasons you shouldn't do what you need to do at the right time.

Think about the Future

Daydreaming can be good when carrying out a task that seems to be stressful to you. For example, while washing the car, especially during the weekend, you can brighten up your mood by thinking about a date you have the next weekend. Think about the things you will say and how you'll dress. Before you realize it, you are through with the task! This approach can be counterproductive if what you're doing requires you to think about it. For example, it isn't advisable when reading your email. However, it's a fantastic way to go through activities that requires your energy and physical strength more than your cognitive ability.

Also, it is vital that you don't let the beautiful thoughts make you stop what you're doing. If you are becoming distracted by the thoughts such that you find yourself resting to focus on the imaginations, you need to find a different method. You can consider listening to music while carrying out the activity. This works well when working out. Create a playlist of your favorite songs and play them while sweating it out.

Leverage your Peak Energy Period

It's not every activity you should do in the morning or in the evening as the case may be. Don't copy the schedule of others because it isn't everything that works for others that will work for you. You need to understand your body to know your peak energy period. Your peak energy period is that part of the day when you're the most energized and alert. For some people, it is in the morning, while it is in the evening for some people. Once you discover your own, you need to reschedule your activities.

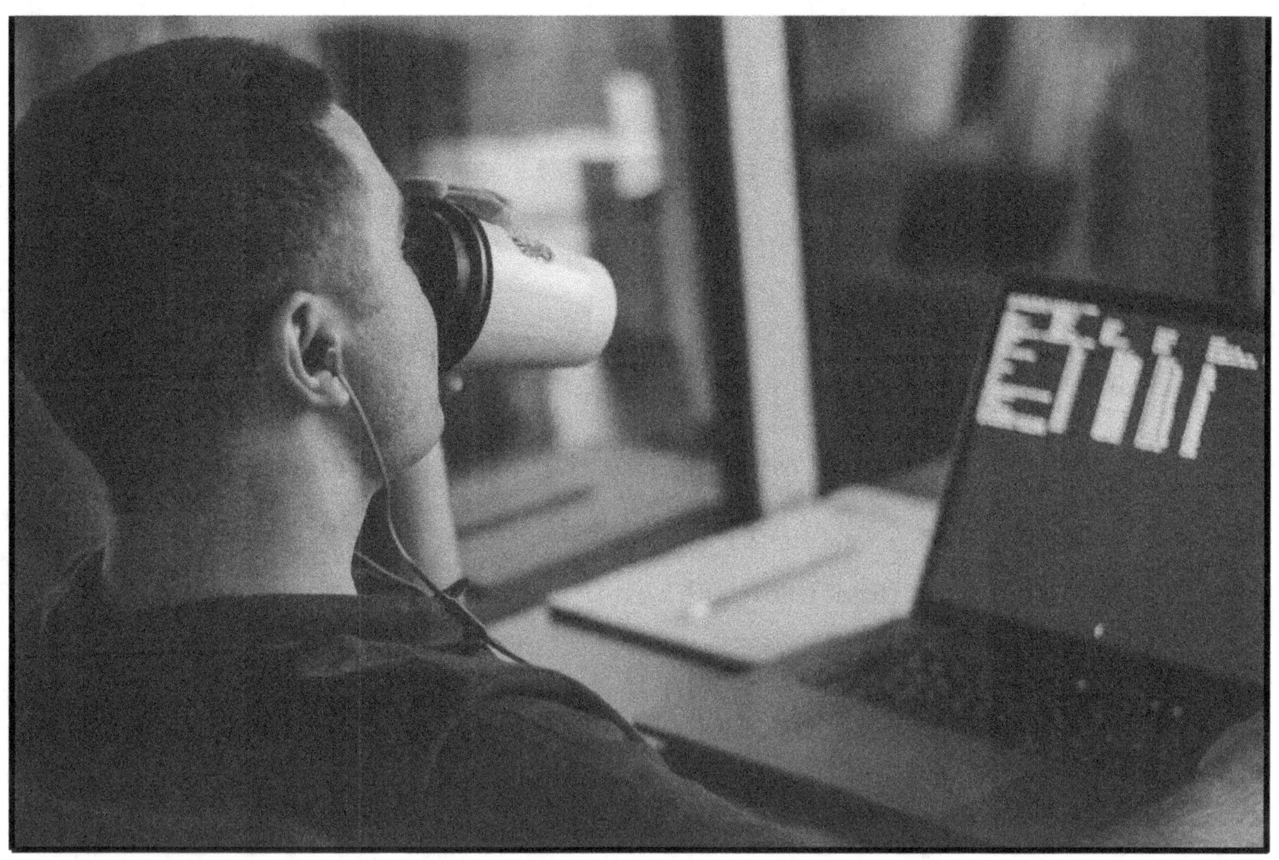

Put those activities that demand more energy and a higher level of alertness in your peak energy period. Move the less demanding ones to the other period of the day. This approach ensures that you'll have enough in the tank for both the demanding and less stressful tasks. You'll no longer end the day feeling that there is more you could have done. You will also stop postponing things you can do today to the next day.

Chapter 5: Health and Fitness Tips

Despite the importance of living healthily, you don't need to spend a lot of money to enjoy it. You only need the right information that'll help you stay healthy and fit. This chapter will highlight and explain some simple but effective health and fitness tips that will improve your experience.

Focus on your Mental Health

One of the reasons people get angry, frustrated, tired, and depressed is prolonged periods of inactivity. On the other hand, active people often feel energetic, experience a better mood, and enjoy a better overall life. So, even if you don't have any reason to be motivated to stay active and participate in an exercise, remembering its impact on your mental health might turn the tide in your favor. Meanwhile, there are many cascading impacts of being mentally healthy, including excellent interpersonal and professional relationships. It also gives you the platform to demonstrate your best ability when you are required to perform.

Start your Day with Exercise

Many people feel discouraged about regular exercise because they assume that it means that they have to hit the gym or run 25 km daily. On the other hand, there are countless lighter activities you can leverage, such as yoga, swimming, walking, and riding a bicycle. In fact, playing with the kids and cleaning up the house is a form of exercise. So, it isn't until you squat double your bodyweight before you can stay active. Start your day with exercise to set you in the right mood for the rest of the day.

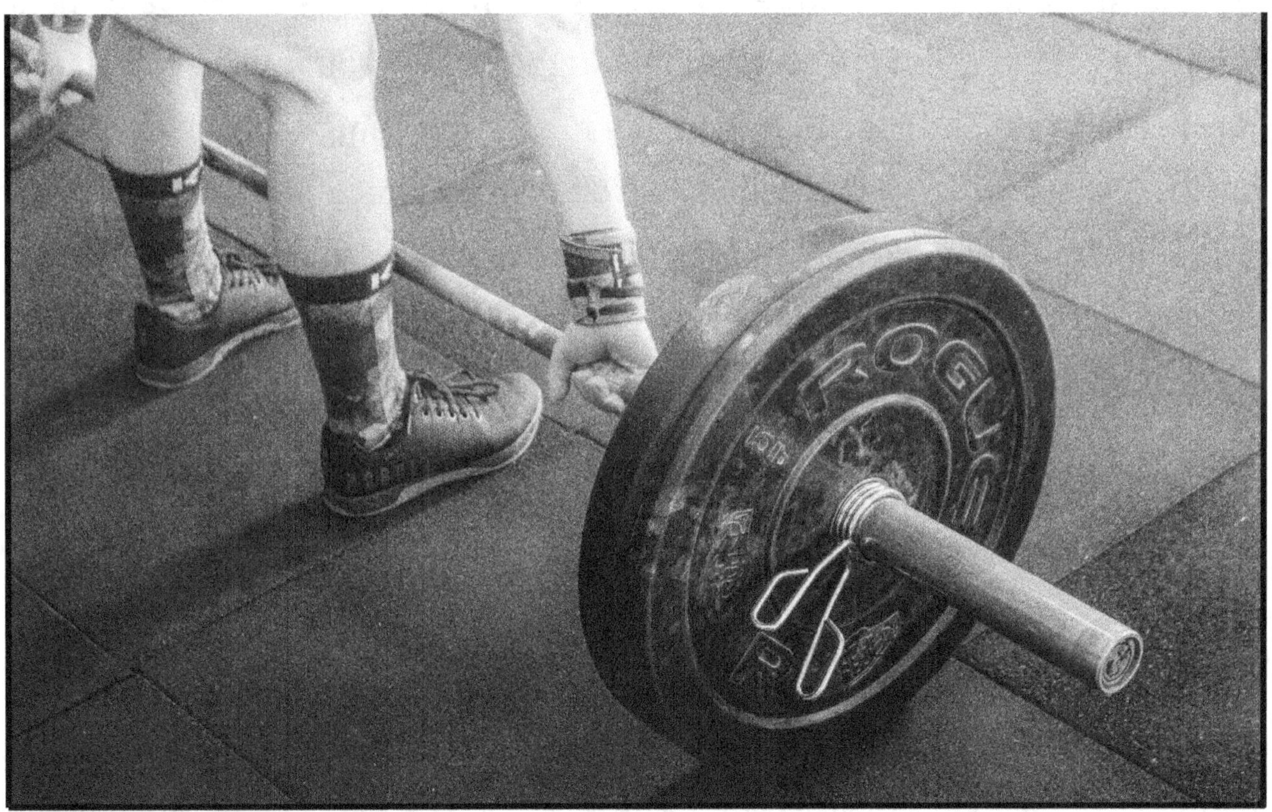

It is recommended that you only do strenuous activities such as sprinting and weightlifting three times a week. At most, it shouldn't be more than five times a week. Let the remaining days be for lighter activity. This approach ensures that you'll be able to continue the routine. Besides, excessive strenuous activities can have negative impacts on your muscles.

Maintain Ideal Mobility and Flexibility Levels

Normally, people in their 20s are supposed to be more flexible. Still, many individuals had lost a lot of flexibility during that period of their lives compared to when they were five years younger. For such people, it is unimaginable to think about how much tighter they would have become in the 40s and 50s. The good news is that you can turn things around if you are having issues with your flexibility. You can enhance the mobility and flexibility levels of your joint as long as you are willing to do it. At least, you should be able to touch your toes. Regular exercise will help you in this regard.

Leverage Flexibility and Mobility Workouts

If you'll be able to improve your mobility and flexibility, you need to take deliberate steps. There are workout routines that can help you in this regard. For example, you can start your workouts with five to ten minutes of stretching. Ensure that you focus more on the tight areas during this exercise. You should also consider doing mobility and flexibility work on the days when you are less busy. This approach will enable you to improve faster and get in the groove quickly whenever you start the workout routine.

Strength Train and Lift Heavy

Studies keep pouring in that prove that strength training, including lifting heavy weights, offers multiple weight benefits. It increases energy levels, maintains weight, and enhances glucose metabolism. Therefore, there are more than enough reasons you should consider strength training. Note that you can use your own kettlebell, dumbbell, barbells, and bodyweight to strength train. Going to a gym can help you because you'll find experts there.

Besides, you will find other people like you that are doing the same thing, and that will inspire and motivate you. Still, you can train in your house if you are focused and disciplined enough. It gets better if you can find a friend that will train with you. You'll challenge yourselves, and the added competition will encourage you to do more. Note that the friend doesn't have to be an expert trainer. As long as he or she is interested in staying fit like you, you have found the right partner.

Check your BMI

The BMI calculator is one of the best ways you can calculate your ideal body weight. Indeed, some people feel that BMI can be misleading. Yet, unless a person possesses unnaturally huge muscles due to steroids, the BMI offers a reasonably accurate calculator of your ideal body weight. You should check it from time to time to evaluate how much weight you have lost or gained during a period. It's not every time that it is obvious that you are gaining or losing pounds. Your mirror might not tell you the true story. Still, you can monitor your ideal weight by checking your BMI.

Keep Healthy Bodyweight and Bodyfat Levels

Diabetes, hypertension, and heart attack are devastating diseases no one wants to contract. However, the reality is that many people in the world today are living with these ailments. One of the risk factors for these illnesses is gaining extra fat. Therefore, you are doing yourself a lot of good when you are involved in activities that can help you maintain healthy bodyfat levels. Note that gaining extra bodyweight in the form of muscle enlargement can also have negative impacts.

Extra weight, whether muscle or fat, has to be carried around by your joints. So, it might start affecting your joint health in the long run, especially when you are growing older. It's in your best interest to avoid gaining excess weight when you're younger to avoid the repercussions in your old age. Stay healthy today for a better future.

Eat Balanced Diets

A balanced diet is a meal that contains all the required nutrients in the right proportion. Our body needs a variety of nutrients to carry out its functions adequately. Note that every food group is needed by the body. You only have to be careful with the quantity you take. Some nutrients are only needed in small amounts. They are called micronutrients, while macronutrients are needed in large quantities by the body. You need to know the ones to eat more and the ones to consume less to maintain your health. For example, you should consume more protein and fewer carbs.

Chapter 6: Healthy Diet Hacks

Everyone wishes to live healthily, but only a few people live in good health. This shows that living healthily is more than wishful thinking. You have to take deliberate steps if you're going to be able to maintain your health. One of the most crucial ways to enjoy good health is by eating healthy diets. This section will highlight and explore some healthy diet hacks that can help you in this regard.

Reduce Carb Intake

Sugars and grains from which fiber and other nutrients have been removed are called refined carbs. Examples include pasta and white flour. These foods are digested quickly and are low in fiber. Therefore, they only keep you full for a short period. You'll soon desire to eat more not long after eating them. Instead of them, choose sources of complex carbohydrates such as oats, veggies like carrots, or ancient grains like barley and quinoa. These options contain more nutrients and will keep you fuller for longer periods.

Shop with a List

Many people are fond of buying unhealthy foods impulsively. You can reduce the chance of doing this by shopping with a list. When you have a list with a specific budget, you'll only buy the things you need. So, it's very likely that you will stick with the healthy items on your list instead of sporadic and unplanned spending.

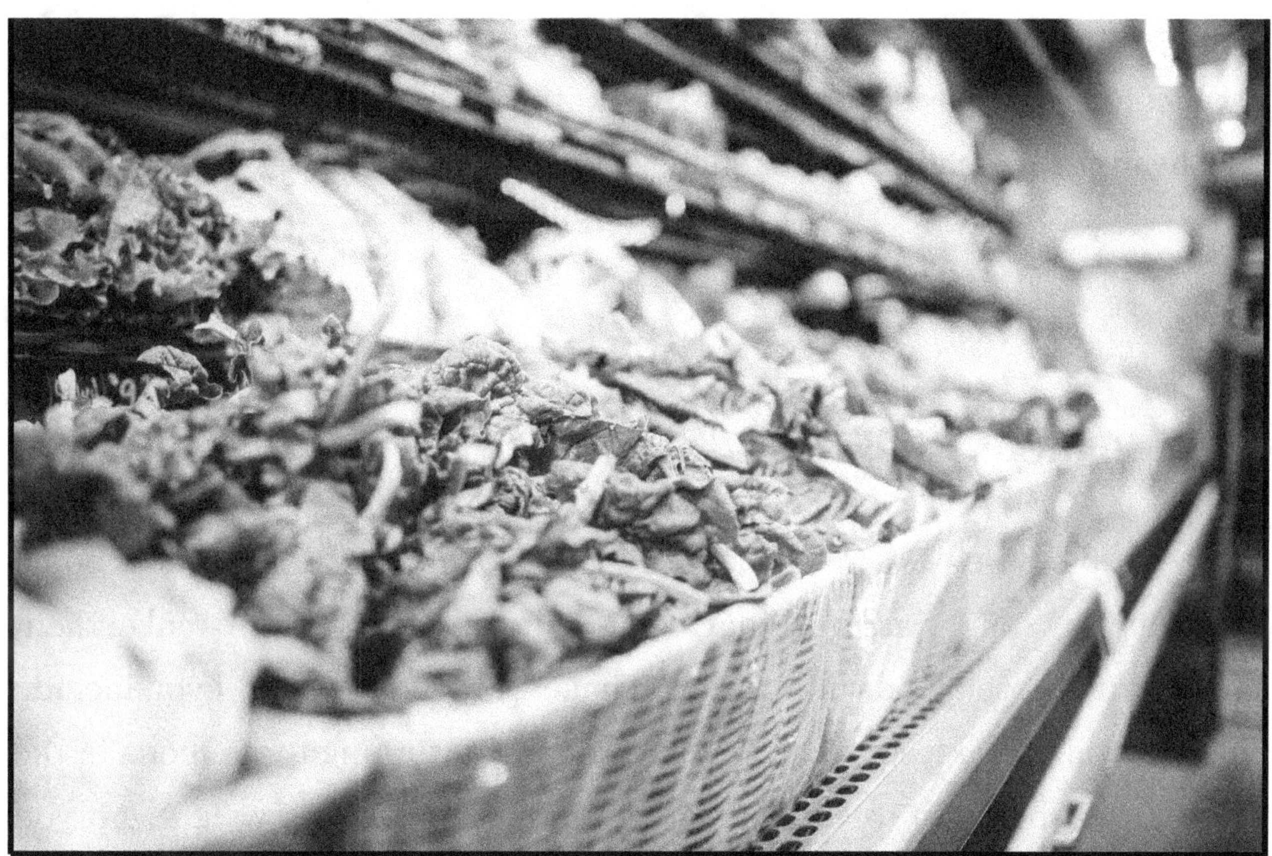

Limit your Consumption of Sodas and Milkshakes

Sodas and milkshakes are renowned for making people gain excess weight. So, it's in your best interest to reduce the way you consume them. Nonetheless, there are less known substances that can have the same effect.

For example, drinks that are advertised for their ability to boost athletic performance can make you put on more weight.

Coffer beverages, sports drinks, and flavored waters are also not safe because they contain excess sugar and artificial colorings. They are often very high in calories, making them risky to your health. Strangely, even juice, which is often promoted as a beneficial beverage, can make you gain weight if you don't control the way you take it. So, hydrating with water is your best bet to stay healthy and maintain your shape.

Have Protein-Rich Breakfasts

Many people have been misled regarding the role of eggs in the body. Some individuals wrongly assume that consuming more eggs will make them fatter. Protein-rich foods like eggs can make a lot of difference if you include them in your breakfast. According to experts, consuming these foods in the morning enables you to stay healthy and cut down excess weight. All you need to do is to swap your daily bowl of cereal for a protein-loaded scramble made with eggs and sautéed vegetables. It is a remarkably effective way to shed pounds.

Consume High-Fiber Foods

Healthy foods such as fruits, vegetables, beans, and whole grains contain fibers. Researchers have discovered that consuming fiber-rich foods will not only help you to lose weight; it will also help you stay in shape. The good news is that adding more fibers to your meal isn't a challenging task. It's as simple as adding beans to your salad, snacking fiber-rich nuts, or eating oats for breakfast.

Eat More Fruits and Vegetables

The nutrients and fibers your body craves are present in vegetables. Besides, investigators have confirmed that consuming vegetables can help you stay healthy and lose weight. Studies have also proven that consuming salad can make you feel full, thereby reducing your craving for more food.

Moreover, scientists have discovered that filling up veggies all day long can help you to maintain a healthy weight. It also reduces the risk of developing diabetes, heart disease, and other chronic diseases. Therefore, it's in your best interest to be more deliberate regarding including vegetables and fruits into your meals daily. The short-term and long-term benefits are worth it when you choose to do it.

Avoid Excess Sugar

Sugar, especially the one for sweet drinks, is one of the major reasons for excess weight gain. It's also linked to health issues such as heart disease and diabetes. Besides, foods like soda, candy, and baked goods contain a lot of added sugars and very low in nutrients needed by the body. It's in your best interest to cut out foods that are high in added sugars because it can help you to lose weight and stay healthy. Note that some organic foods can be incredibly high in sugar. Therefore, endeavor to read nutrition labels before consuming any food.

Consume More Healthy Fats

It is common to make fat the first thing you want to reduce when trying to lose weight. Yet, healthy fats can actually help you to slim down. In fact, several studies have proven that a high-fat diet that has food such as avocados, olive oil, and nuts can help to optimize weight loss. Besides, fats make you feel fuller, thereby reducing the craving for more food. So, consuming healthy fats can help you to stay on track while maintaining your weight and health.

Eat More Home-Made Foods

If you know how to cook, you have a skill that can help you eat healthily and avoid gaining excess weight. Research has proven that home-made meals help you to stay healthy and promote weight loss. There's no doubt that you will have a great time when you eat at a nice restaurant. However, restaurants are set up to scintillate your taste bud rather than keep you healthy.

Therefore, you are doing yourself a lot of good by cooking your meals. You'll have control over the choice of ingredients, allowing you to choose healthy ones that will enable you to prioritize your health. Besides, it helps you to save more money, especially if you are on a relatively low budget.

Walk More

Your automobile is meant to be a blessing that will cut down your stress level. Nonetheless, if you're not careful, you might get used to it and become lazy. You don't have to drive everywhere. Walk when the distance isn't too far to exercise your muscles. Walking is a fantastic way to lose weight without going through strenuous routines. According to scientists, thirty minutes of walking per day can help you lose weight tremendously in the long run. Moreover, it's an effortless and enjoyable activity you can have indoors or outdoors.

Focus on your Food When Eating

When consuming food without thinking about what you're doing, you will not get the best out of the experience. Still, that's not the only problem. Another issue that comes with being distracted when you're eating is that you might consume more calories than required, leading to weight gain. So, avoid eating while watching a movie or sitting with your computer. Eat at the dining table so that you can have control over the quantity you're consuming. Scrolling through emails on your smartphone while eating is also a habit you should discard to ensure that you concentrate on your meal.

Chapter 7: How to Get More Quality Sleep

The sleep process and its benefits deserve a complete book. Sleep is one of the most important processes of the body that offers numerous advantages. Getting quality sleep is a habit you shouldn't handle with levity. In this section, we will explore the benefits of getting restorative sleep and how you can improve your sleeping habit.

Benefits of Restorative Sleeps

Below are some of the perks that come with good sleeping habits:

Peak Energy Levels

Many processes are taking place in your body when you're sleeping. For example, many repair and maintenance works occur in the body during the sleep period. Your body needs you to be inactive so that it can carry out its tasks without interference. You need to give it enough time to perform these functions. If not, you'll wake up feeling jaded and tired. However, when you sleep on time, you'll feel like your "battery" has been fully recharged.

Consequently, you'll have enough energy to carry out your activities during the day.

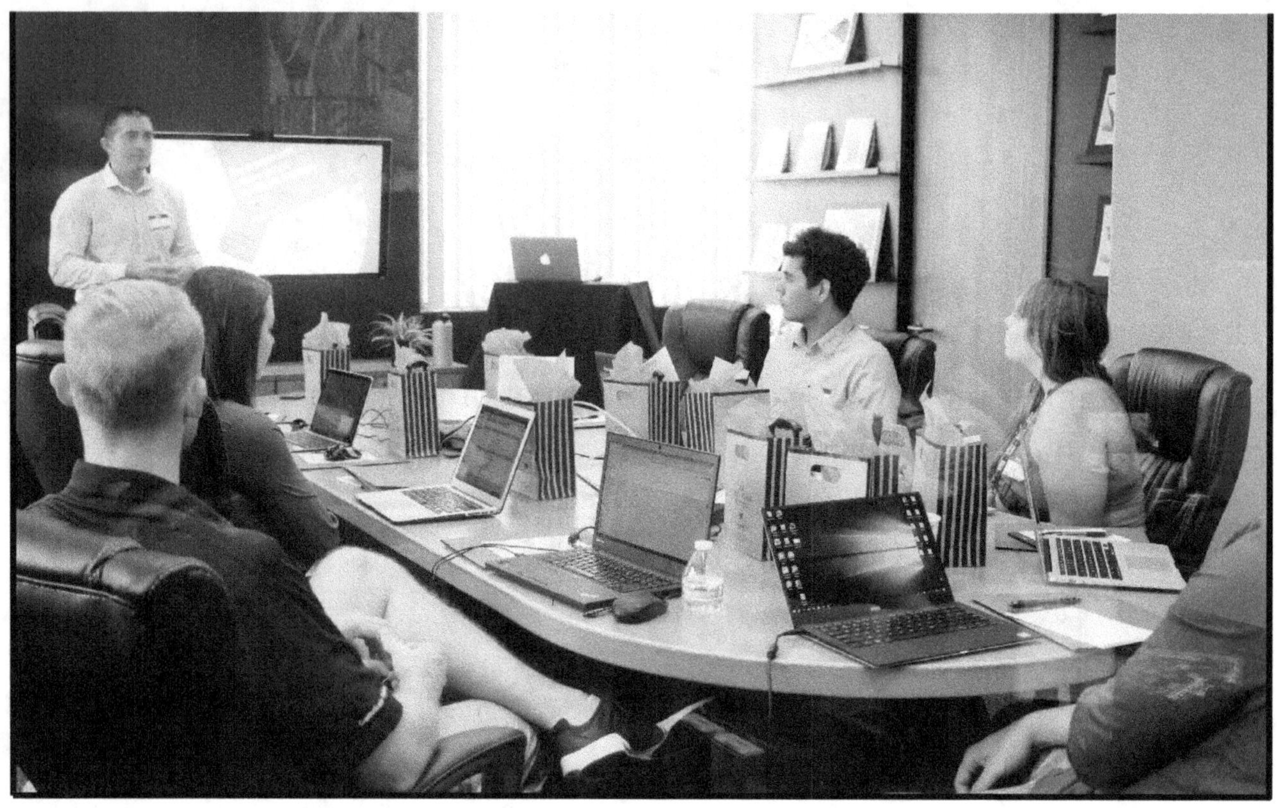

Enhanced Performance

Peak energy levels are the bedrock of fantastic performances. When you didn't sleep well, you'll feel tired and stressed, which can impede your preparation and eventual performance. It gets worse and obvious when you're involved in mentally challenging activities such as writing and data analysis. You might struggle to come up with creative ideas, which can be frustrating. Whenever you have a crucial interview or presentation, ensure you're well-rested to give yourself the platform to perform at your best.

Feeling of Contentment

Unknown to many, your sleep habit can affect your psychological health. One of the reasons some people feel disgruntled during the day and feel like life isn't worth it is because they didn't sleep well. When you start your day on the wrong note due to poor sleeping habits, you'll find it hard to get into the groove during the day. You'll not perform as expected, and you can start feeling frustrated about your life. It can affect your reactions to others, further compounding your woes.

Quality Interpersonal Relationships

Failure to sleep well can make you wake up in the wrong mood. Meanwhile, when you are disgruntled, you're not likely to give good responses to your friends and family. Indeed, some people are emotionally intelligent enough to control their feelings and relate well. Yet, some people find it difficult to say the right things when they feel exhausted.

Remember that negative responses can cause fracas that cannot be mended between you and your loved ones. So, it is in your best interest to have a restorative sleep so that you can "wake up on the right side of your bed". If you notice that you are arguing more with friends and families, you need to relax more and improve your sleeping habit.

Enhancement of Immune System

The body has its own "soldiers" that protect it against germ invaders. These fighters are part of a system of the body called the immune system. When this system is at its peak powers, it is going to be very difficult for any disease to attack your body. However, once it is weak, your body becomes susceptible to infections.

So, whatever boosts this system will help you to keep the doctor away. Thankfully, scientists have discovered that a good sleeping habit is an immune booster. This discovery was made by investigators of the American Academy of Sleep Medicine. In fact, the researcher claims that quality sleep makes vaccines more effective.

Quality Professional Relationships

Due to your calmness, emotional intelligence, and optimum performance at work, because you're sleeping well, you will enhance your professional relationships. You'll find it easier to get along well with both your employers and your colleagues when you're well-rested.

Tips for Getting Better Sleep

You can improve the quality of your sleep by leveraging the following tips.

Have a Regular Bedtime and Wake-up Time

Your body has a way of adjusting to your habits to increase efficiency and save energy. If you don't have a specific sleep and wake up-time, your body's circadian rhythm will be disrupted, and this will affect you. This is one of the reasons you'll notice that you slept but woke up feeling tired. Set specific times and let your body get into the groove. It might take a week or two, but once your body gets used to it, you'll feel more energized after sleeping.

Avoid Using Bright Lights in your Room

When you're exposed to the sunshine in the morning, your body soaks it up, and you'll feel rejuvenated. The boost in energy enables you to complete tasks faster and more effectively. When the sun sets, you should avoid bright lights because your body will assume that it's still daylight and want to stay alert and active. This exposure can prevent you from sleeping on time. So, it is in your best interest to ensure that your room is dark to lull your body to sleep on time.

Let your Bed only be for Sleeping

Many people have a practice of doing different activities when they are in bed at night, such as reading, watching TV, and pressing their phones. If you know that you're not ready to sleep, don't get into your bed. Your body might adjust to your refusal to sleep on the bed and start getting alert instead of sleeping. So, use other places for other activities at night. Once you jump on your bed, your body should know that it is time to sleep.

Avoid Napping during the Day

It's natural that you feel tired and sleepy sometimes during the day. Nevertheless, you need to be careful with the way you do it so that you won't set the wrong precedence for your body. Don't take a nap unless you are sick because it will disrupt your sleep at night. If you must sleep, ensure that it's up to fifteen to twenty minutes. Even if you have to do that, let it be in the late afternoon. Sleeping during the evenings will prevent you from sleeping on time at night.

Wind Down Late in the Day

Try as much as possible to avoid taking your stressors to bed with you. One of the easiest ways you can achieve this is by doing all your strenuous activities in the day. Wind down towards the end of the day to ease yourself to sleep. When you do strenuous tasks before you sleep, you'll fall asleep out of exhaustion, which isn't beneficial to your body. Such sleep can make you wake up with a headache. Instead, do lighter tasks so that you can slow down until you eventually sleep to feel refreshed when you wake up.

Have a Bedtime Routine

Your body craves routines that it can follow consistently. You can take advantage of this fact to teach your body how to sleep on time. Have things you do when you are about to sleep. For example, you can take a warm bath before bedtime or listen to your favorite song or playlist. Once your body gets used to the routine, it'll start preparing to sleep once you initiate the ritual. Ensure that it is consistent to get the best results.

Chapter 8: Benefits of Drinking More Water

There is no doubt that drinking water is an essential and beneficial habit. It helps to ensure that we don't choke when we eat. Yet, there are more perks to enjoy when you drink a lot of water. Here are other advantages of drinking more water.

Joint Lubrication

Cartilages are present in joints and discs of the spine. Interestingly, they contain 80% water. So, long-term dehydration can reduce the shock-absorbing ability of the joints. This is one of the reasons people experience joint pain. Scientists have discovered long ago that the human body is like a machine with various parts carrying out specific operations.

Just like cars, our bodies need to be maintained to ensure that they keep functioning at optimum levels. Water does the same thing engine oils do in a machine. They lubricate the joint by hydrating the cartilages. Therefore, one of the ways you can ensure that you avoid joint pain is by drinking more water. This relatively cheap and easy habit can save you the cost of getting an appointment with a doctor later.

Formation of Saliva and Mucus

You need saliva to aid the digestion process. Besides, it is crucial to ensure that your nose, mouth, and eyes are moist. The benefit of keeping these body parts moist is that it prevents friction and damage to them. When you drink more water, you are also keeping your mouth clean. Moreover, you cannot wash your mouth without using water.

Sweets and candy are sumptuous, but they can lead to tooth decay. We can hardly avoid them because they are given to us on special occasions. Still, it is crucial to limit their impact on our dental set. Drinking more water can help you to avoid tooth decay. Choosing water above sweetened beverages can also help in this regard.

Reduction in Chance of a Hangover

The list of the side effects of excessive consumption of alcohol is endless. There are short-term and long-term negatives impacts of taking this depressant. One of the short-term effects is a hangover. A hangover is that undesirable physical condition following the heavy consumption of alcohol. It is often characterized by nausea and headache.

People often experience this effect in the morning after heavy drinking the previous night. It can be avoided by alternating alcoholic drinks with unsweetened soda water, ice, and lemon when partying. Don't let the enjoyment of the moment make you damn the terrible consequences the following day.

Weight Loss

There is a lot of pressure for many people to lose weight today because of the prevalence of subtle or obvious body-shaming jabs at plus-size people. Nonetheless, there are many benefits of losing weight apart from getting a dream physique. It staves off obesity and its negative impacts. So, you can choose to lose weight for the right reasons.

If that is the case, there are many effective ways to go about it. Thankfully, there are even free ways to do it. One of the cheap and easy methods of losing weight that many people ignore is the consumption of more water. Drinking water before eating will make you consume less food because you will quickly have a sense of fullness.

Enhances Performance During Exercise

Sportspeople have a culture of taking water breaks. It is not a futile activity. They do this because it boosts their performance. According to experts, drinking more water enhances performance, especially during strenuous activities. Indeed, more studies are needed to confirm this suggestion. Yet, there is evidence that this claim might not be far from the truth.

For example, a review discovered that dehydration impedes performance, especially when an activity lasts longer than thirty minutes. One of the reasons you tire easily during the day might be because you have not been drinking enough water. You can turn this negative pattern around by consuming more fluid.

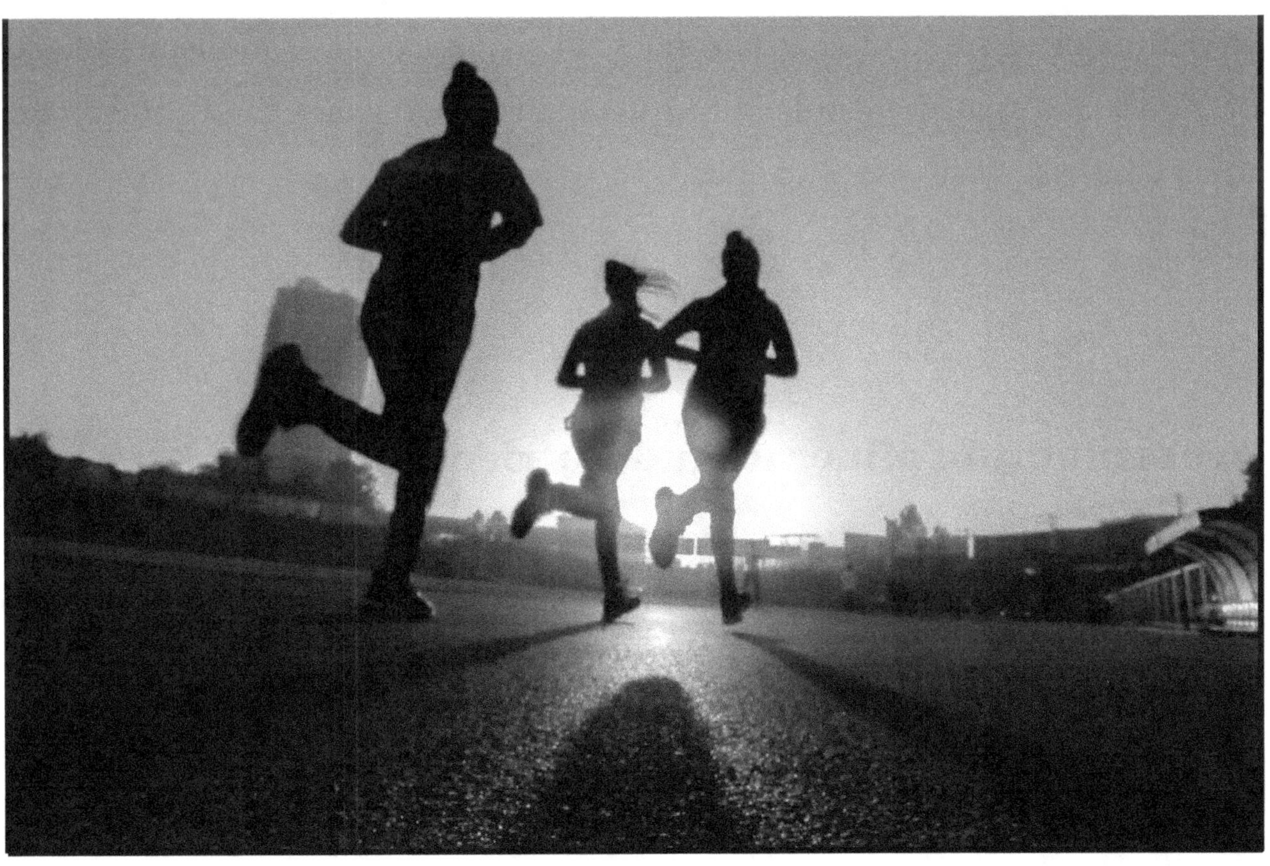

Prevention of Kidney Damage

Water helps to make minerals more accessible to the body by dissolving them. It also aids the removal of waste products. Consequently, water is essential to the functioning and maintenance of the kidney. The kidney filters close to 120-150 quarts of fluid daily. Approximately 1-2 quarts of this amount are removed in the form of urine from the body while the bloodstream recovers the rest. Drinking plenty water helps to reduce the risk of developing Urinary tract infections.

Kidney stones are another disease you can prevent by drinking water. People battling this health condition were diagnosed after they didn't take the required amount of water per day. Note that people dealing with kidney stones are often susceptible to chronic kidney disease. The American College of Physicians issued a guideline in 2014 that increasing fluid intake can reduce the risk of stone recurrence.

Accessibility of Minerals and Nutrients

Taking supplements and healthy meals are meant to help you boost the functioning of your body. However, that purpose will be defeated when these nutrients and minerals aren't accessible to the organs and tissues that need them. Lack of adequate fluid is one of the reasons the body is unable to get what it needs.

Water dissolves minerals in the body, thereby making them accessible to the body parts that need them. Note that around 60% of the body contains water. So, the more water you take, the more you are increasing the chances of circulating necessary nutrients and minerals all over the body.

Supports the Airways

The human body is an intelligent system. It makes decisions that it feels are best for it, and you need to understand this process to increase your chances of living healthily. For example, if your body realizes that it doesn't have enough water, it will make moves to manage what it has. One of the ways it does this is by restricting the airways.

Apparently, this move is dangerous because you will struggle to breathe well. This will make things worse for people suffering from asthma and other allergies. Therefore, you should consume more water to prevent your body from making drastic decisions that can affect your airways.

Maintenance of Blood Pressure

The last thing you want is high or low blood pressure. Without normal blood pressure, blood will not flow around the circulatory system appropriately. When this occurs, your body won't be able to get the nutrient and oxygen it needs to carry out its activities. Your body will also lack white blood cells and antibodies that protect it against invading germs.

The fresh blood that is delivered to the organs also helps to pick up toxic wastes and products of metabolism. When you don't drink enough water, your blood can become thicker. Once this happens, it will increase your blood pressure, which can lead to cardiac arrest.

Regulation of Body Temperature

When your body heats up, water stored in the skin's middle layers comes to the surface of the skin as sweat. The body cools down as the water evaporate, especially during exercise. Scientists believe that the body will struggle to tolerate heat strain when there is too little water in the body. Heat storage will increase, and it will become difficult for the body to regulate its temperature.

So, you need to help your body by drinking more water. Drinking more water will reduce physical strain on the body when heat stress occurs during exercise. When the body is unable to regulate its temperature, you may need to see the doctor soon.

Conclusion

In reality, nothing is certain in life. Still, we can make plans and carry out activities that can give us a higher chance of living fuller and more meaningful lives. Healthy habits are some of those things in life that increase our chances of making the most of our experiences in the world. No one wants to be sick. However, a wish is not enough. You need to take deliberate steps that will boost your chances of keeping the doctor away.

You have been exposed to many tips and hacks that can help you boost your physical and mental health in this book. Take advantage of them to improve the quality of your life. Nothing good comes easy, and you need to be resolute and disciplined to continue on this path of healthy living. Remember that life is too short to be lived in pain and agony. So, invest in your health because that is all you have got. If you lose it, no amount of money or awards can replace it.

Only a healthy person can enjoy the fruits of his or her labor. So, while striving to get to the top of your career, don't neglect your health. Whatever career path you choose that is making it impossible to prioritize your physical and mental health is not worth it. You deserve to be happy and healthy. However, you can never experience the beauty of life when you sacrifice your health and happiness for honors. That is too much of a sacrifice. Start inculcating the healthy habits you have learned in this book to make the most of your experience in life.